Cupping Therapy

(A Therapeutic Traditional Regimen)

By

Malik IH MD (PSM)
Rajiv Gandhi University, Bangalore
India

CS Independent Publishing Platform, South Carolina, North Charleston, USA

Book Details

Paperback: 119 pages
Publisher: CS Independent Publishing Platform; 2nd edition (Octoberr, 2015)
Language: English
ISBN-10: 1518762875
ISBN-13: 978-1518762871
Product Dimensions: 6 x 9 inches

Corresponding email: izhunaz@gmail.com

Contact: 91-8287833547
Cupping Therapy
First Edition: 2014, Second Ed 2015
Publisher: CS Independent Publishing Platform; 2nd edition

Notice

Knowledge and practice in medical field are constantly changing. As new research and experience broaden our knowledge simultaneously present treatment trends are becoming dangerous rather than solving the ailments due to their unavoidable side-effects, people are looking for alternative like cupping therapy. Medical experts are advising and luring towards this basic and effective alternative and traditional therapy (cupping therapy). Changes in practice, treatment and cupping procedures may become necessary or appropriate. Readers are advised to check the most current information provided on procedures advised, administered/applied, verify the recommendation for therapy, the method and duration of application and contraindications. It is the responsibility of the practitioner, relying on their own experience and knowledge of the patient, to make diagnoses, to determine indications and the best treatment for each individual patient according to basic concepts of treatment and to take all appropriate safety precautions. To the fullest extent of the law, neither the Publisher nor the Author assumes any liability for any injury and/or damage to persons or property arising out or related to any use of the material or procedure contained in this book.

Malik IH

About the book

Blood letting is an ancient medical procedure comprises of wet cupping, leeching, and Venesection; still in use across the world. The evidence of cupping therapy for blood letting procedure can be traced back in ancient system of medicine like Greco-roman, Indian and Arabic medicine. Now a days cupping therapy is an established therapeutic modality among Indian system of medicine (*Unani* and Ayurveda) as well as worldwide. Inspite of that, standard operative procedure (SOPs) for cupping therapy is yet to develop. In this book author comprises the possible indications of cupping therapy along with procedures, application points, safety concerns, historical perspective, surgical operative standards, and contraindication of the same described in *traditional* system of medicine.

This book is doctor-friendly because it would help the alternative medical practitioners involved in providing not only curative services, but also preventive and promotive services to the community at large, motivating them to a healthier, and happier life.

Despite my sincere efforts to make the book accurate and comprehensive as I could, it is possible there may be some gaps or errors in the book. I would be most grateful to the readers, if these deficiencies are pointed out so that can be removed in the next edition. I also invite healthy suggestions from all readers to help us improve the quality of book and achieve the purpose with which it has been written. All such feedback would be carefully considered and gratefully acknowledged.

Malik IH

"If we all treat each other like we treat ourselves what a wonderful place earth would be"

INDEX

Cupping therapy

Since ancient times, complementary and alternative medicine (CAM) have played an important role in human health and welfare. Many therapeutic approaches in healthcare outside the realm of conventional medicine persist in various parts of the world. There is considerable scientific and commercial potential in CAM, which needs to be explored precisely. Cupping therapy is practiced across the world. Cupping involves applying a heated cup to generate a partial vacuum that mobilizes the blood flow and promotes effective healing. This review outlines various tools and techniques of cupping therapy.

In Arabic they say, "A certain person diminished the problem", they meant that he returned the problem to its original size. There is also a verb "ahjama" which means "to withdraw or retreat from attack". Thus he who performed the cupping operation made diseases refrain from attacking him. The increase of spoiled blood in the body rendered its cessation from growing when the person became twenty-two years old, and it accumulated in the back area of the person. With advance in age, these accumulations of spoiled blood hindered the circulation of the whole blood, eventually paralyzed the work of the young red corpuscles then the body became weak and exposed to various kinds of diseases. When one performed cupping, the blood returned to its original condition and the stagnant blood went away (that blood which contained maximum rate of senile red corpuscles and their cells ghosts and abnormal shapes of red blood cells, and other impurities). The pressure on the blood circulation was lessened and the pure blood formed from young red corpuscles rushed to feed the cells and the body organs, and released them from harmful residues, damages and unwanted materials. Al'lah's envoy "Mohammed" (Communication with Al' lah and Peace are through him) said, "Cupping is the most helpful act for human beings to cure themselves with." [1,31]

CUPPING, HISTORICAL BACKGROUND

There are numerous reports mentioned in the history including Herodotus (a Greek historian, 400 BC) prescription related to wet and dry Cupping therapy for treatment of headaches, lack of appetite, maldigestion, fainting, abscess evacuation, narcolepsy, and others.[1] It also finds a mention in the famous Egyptian Papyrus Ebers (1550 BC) in the west and ancient Greek medicine. Hippocrates (Greece) preached the cupping based treatments related with musculoskeletal diseases of the back and extremities, gynecological complaints, pharyngitis, ear ailments, and lung diseases. Cupping therapy is popular as 'Al-Hijama' in Egypt and Arabic countries. It is an intervention of Asian medicinal systems such as Unani,

Ayurveda, Chinese, Tibetan, and Oriental Medicine in Asia, the Middle East, and European countries. In Europe, cupping therapy was customarily used by monastery practitioners and folk healers up to the 19th century. [2, 3, 4, 5, 6, 7] Scientist Celsus advised local cupping for abscesses and as a means of extracting poisons from bites made by man, apes, dogs, wild animals or snakes. In the early 2nd century, scientist Aretaeus used both wet and dry cupping, but preferred the former to treat prolapse of the uterus and cholera ileus and epilepsy. Galen was a great proponent of the method and described various cups of glass, horn, and brass. [8] Horn cupping and bamboo jar therapy were derived from cupping therapy principles. [9] Dry and wet cupping are commonly practiced in the Far

East, Middle East, and Eastern Europe as well. [10-30] Thus, cupping therapy maintains a strong historical account that needs to be rejuvenated in modern times.

The use of cupping therapy is documented in the history of most great cultures and civilisations of the past with the earliest available records revealing extensive use by the ancient Egyptians, Chinese and Middle Eastern cultures. In the west, cupping therapy was part of the basic repertoire of clinical skills a doctor would be expected to understand and practice until the latter part of the 19th century. In parts of Western Europe there has been a recent upsurge in the interest from both public and academic perspectives. Scientific studies have began researching the effects of cupping therapy in an attempt to better understand the mechanisms underpinning this fascinating medical treatment that has truly withstood the test of time. Celebrity endorsements by professional sports players, celebrities, and seniorinternational politicians.[10-13]

METHODS OF CUPPING THERAPY

Cupping therapy belongs to a 2000-year-old Chinese traditional medicine system. There are 10 types of different cupping methods viz. weak/light cupping, medium cupping, strong cupping, moving cupping, needle cupping, moxa/hot needle cupping, empty/flash cupping, full/bleeding cupping, herbal cupping, and water cupping.[11] Traditionally, cups were made of glass, metals or even bamboo.[12] A gourd was explored as the medium for cupping by ancient Greeks.[1] Since these traditional cups do not allow the complete cupping of big joints, a modern technology of pulsatile cupping was developed that generates a pulsatile vacuum for complete cupping. Silicone cups allow comprehensive cupping of big joints

16

along with flexibility in therapy.[1, 12] Different shapes of cups are available from balls to bells in variable sizes, ranging from 25–75 mm across the opening.[13] Across the world, different types of cups are available for cupping which are listed in Table 1.[14]

Table 1.

Types of cups explored for cupping therapy and their origin.

Cups	Region
Round glass cups or bell shape cups	Japan
Buffalo horn shape cups	North America
Hollow animal horn shape cups	Europe, Asia, Africa, and North America

Cups	Region
Mouth or buffalo horn shape cups	Iraq to the Mediterranean (Assyrian Empire period)
Shell shape cups	North America (specifically near Vancouver Island)

Based on the application of cups, cupping therapies are classified and described as inFig. 1.[7, 15]

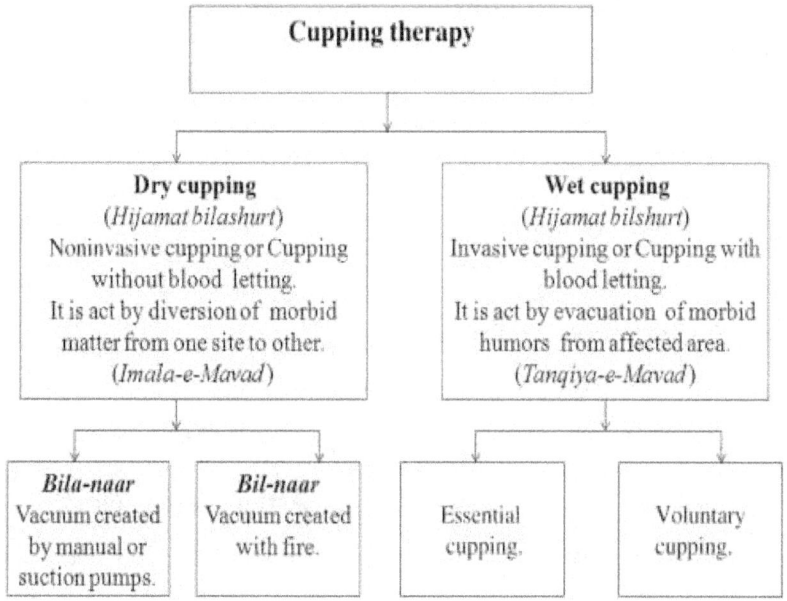

Fig. 1. Classification of cupping therapies.

It is the most commonly used method in traditional and Chinese medicine wherein suction is generated by use of a flame. Dry cupping is a technique of bruising the skin painlessly, in which the bottom of a glass cup is rinsed with methylated spirits, set alight, and planted over the skin. The flame exhausts the supply of oxygen, causing a partial vacuum and the skin is sucked into the mouth of the glass. Retained cupping is utilized to stimulate mammary glands for improving milk ejection. It also assists in healing of wounds via quick pus discharge.[15,16] It contains two steps: (1) prior to the application of suction, small incisions are made with a triangle-edged or plum-blossom needle to the cups; and (2) an acupoint is firmly tapped for a short time to cause bleeding. In the case of wet cupping, prophetic medicine, honey is applied locally to fix the cups, as well as for the skin scarification, hence enhancing the rate of healing.[17] Wet cupping involves two different application methodologies, viz. cupping, puncturing and cupping (CPC) method. CPC progressed with six steps of skin demarcation, sterilization, cupping, puncturing, cupping, and sterilization. This method is commonly use in Arabic nations[18,19] to treat the various disease conditions. The puncturing and cupping (PC) method followed five steps of skin demarcation, sterilization, puncturing, cupping, and sterilization. The PC method is common in China, Korea, and Germany.[20, 21] In this method, practitioners need to control the suction by gently moving the cup in one direction.[22] On comparing the cupping across the meridian running direction and that against the running direction, similar local effects were observed. Dual-directional moving cupping is applicable for the treatment of local disorders. The abscopal effect is better with moving the cup against the meridian running direction.2[3] When cups are removed after suction without delay, then it is called empty cupping.[22]

In needle cupping, acupuncture is applied initially with subsequent deposition of cups over the needle. Medicinal/herbal cupping makes exclusive use of bamboo cups wherein the herbs are boiled as aqueous dispersions followed by application of suction on specific points.[22] The acupuncture method merged with cupping works by the following mechanism – small needles inserted into the skin will contact tension points and thereby relieve the pain. It is widely accepted as a safe therapy, even though the probability of complications such as trauma or infection persists.[24] The length of needle retreat in cupping depends on the patient gender and the negative pressure of cupping.[25] Water cupping comprised filling a glass or bamboo cup with one third warm water and pursuing the cupping process in a rather quick fashion.[22]

Each kind of cupping therapy finds uses in different ailments. Since cupping is widely used in Chinese folklore culture, the technique has been inherited by the modern Chinese practitioners. In cupping, the heating power of flames aids in achieving suction (negative pressure) inside the cups which have to be employed on the desired part of the body.[22] In sham cupping, a small hole to reduce the negative pressure after suction aids in maintaining the inner pressure for real cupping therapy, but yet more rigorous research calls for safe use of this device.[26] Sliding cupping involves three steps viz. (1) the local area of pain, or the affected channels and points are lubricated; (2) the cup is applied; and (3) the cup is made to slide up and down until the skin becomes hyperemic. This is known to resolve the disturbed functions of Zang-fu via a dual mechanism of cupping as well as massage. Zang-fu is a collective term for internal organs; five zang organs encompass the heart, liver, spleen, lungs, and kidneys and the six fu organs contain gallbladder, stomach, small intestine, large intestine, urinary bladder, and sanjiao (the triple energizer). [27] El Sayed et al described cupping therapy in the form of 'S' techniques, as depicted in Fig. 2. [28]

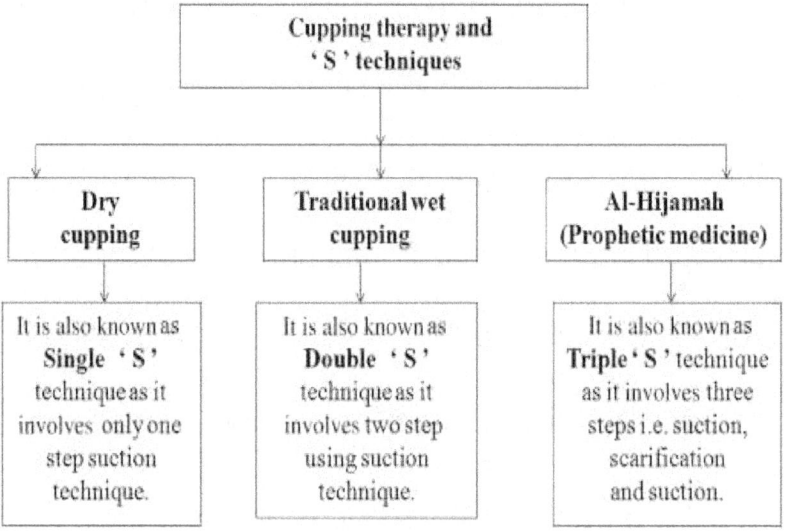

Fig. 2. Cupping therapy and 'S' techniques

APPLICATION SITES FOR CUPPING

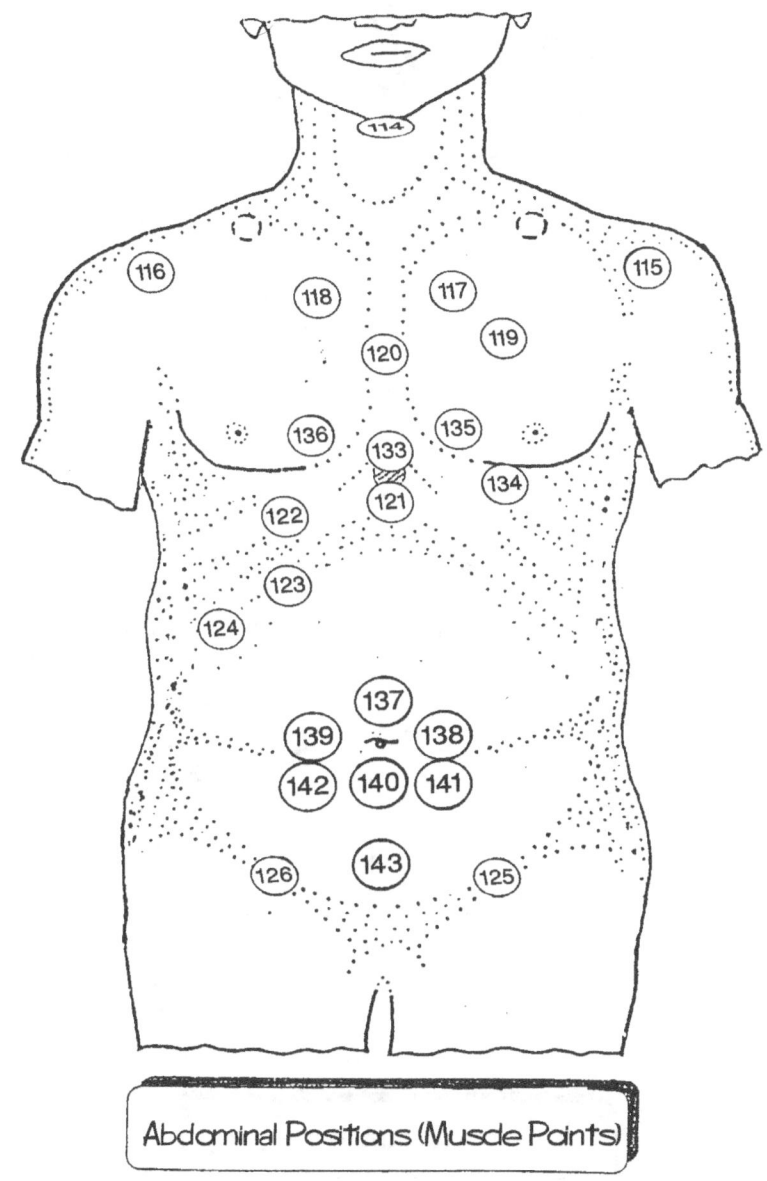

Abdominal Positions (Muscle Points)

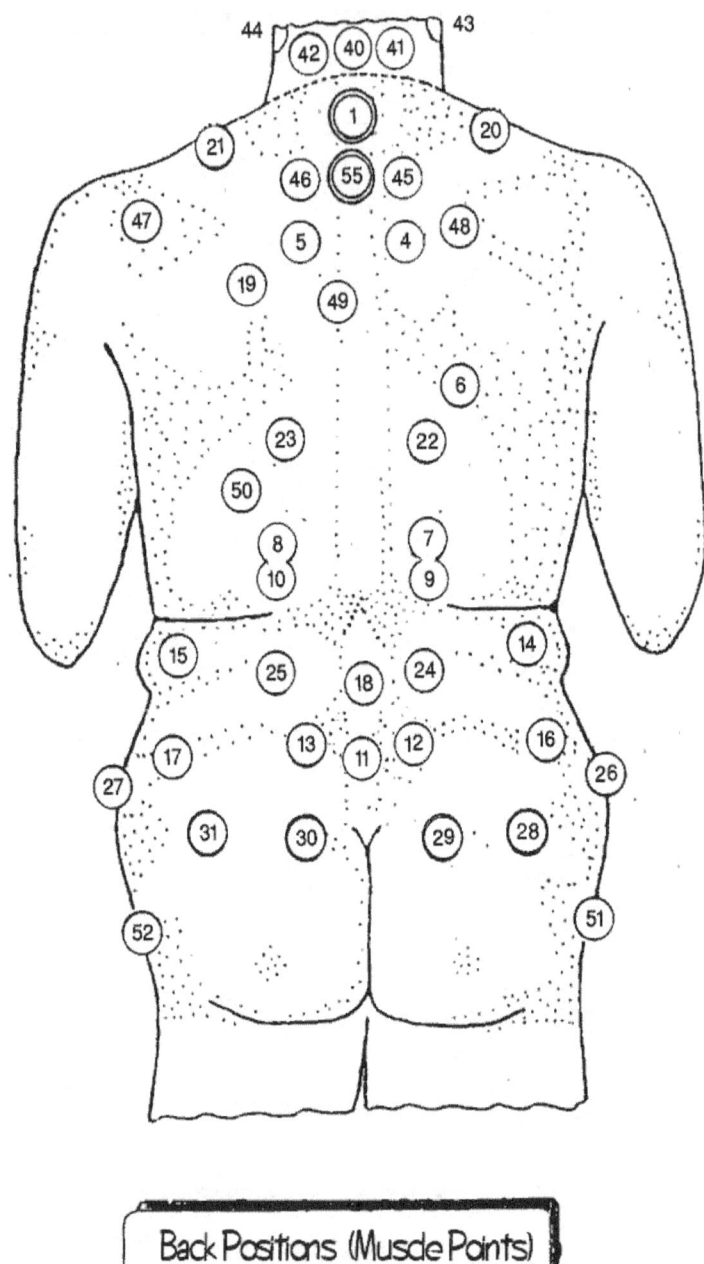

Back Positions (Muscle Points)

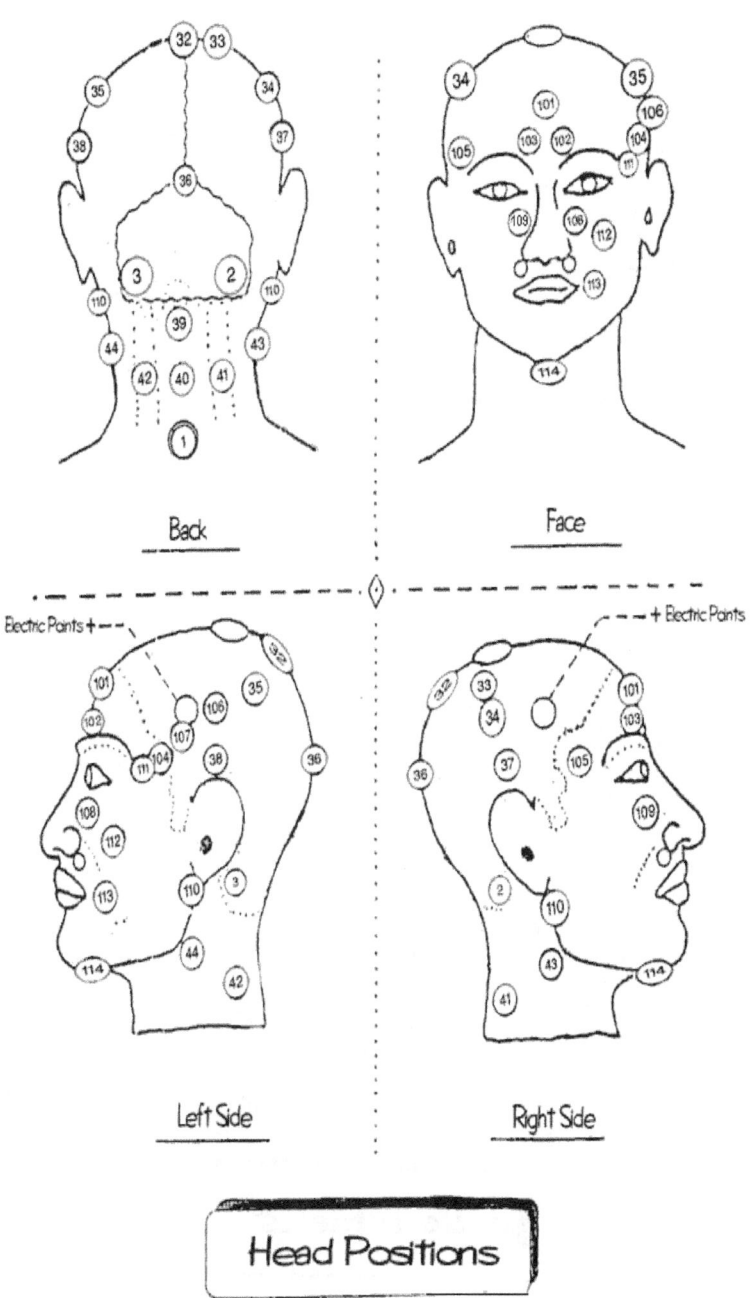

Back

Face

Electric Points +

+ Electric Points

Left Side

Right Side

Head Positions

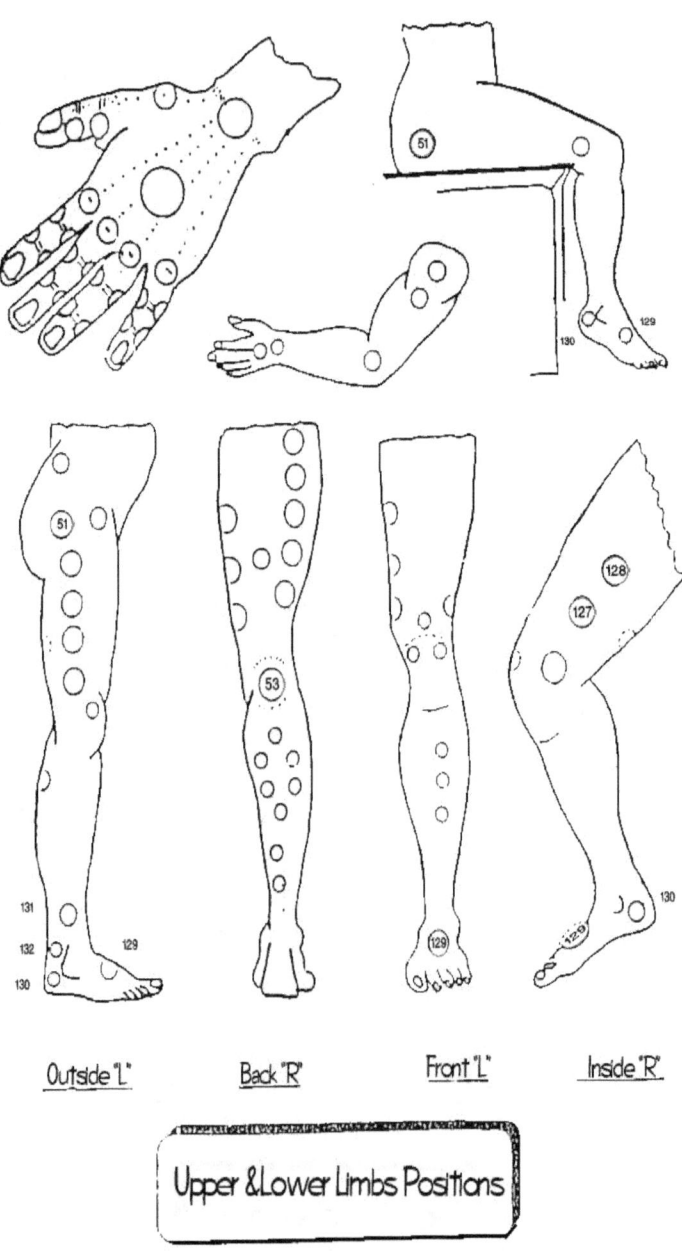

Outside "L"   Back "R"   Front "L"   Inside "R"

Upper & Lower Limbs Positions

Group (A)[29]

- **Rheumatism (painful joints)** (points 1, 55, in addition to all areas of pain).

- **Roughness of knee** (points 1, 55, 11, 12, 13 and cupping around the knee and you may add 53, 54).

- **Oedema (swollen tissue due to build up of fluid)** (points 1, 55, 130, the right and left side of the heel and you may add 9, 10).

- **Sciatic pain (nerve pain from the buttock which goes down the leg)** (for the right leg) (points 1, 55, 11, 12, 26, 51 and places of pain on the leg especially the beginning and the end of the muscle) (for the left leg) (points 1, 55, 11, 13, 27, 52 and places of pain on the leg especially the beginning and the end of the muscle).

- **Back pain** (positions 1, 55 and cupping on both sides of the spine and places of pain).

- **Neck/shoulder pain** (points 1, 55, 40, 20, 21 and places of pain).

- **Gout (swollen joints due to excess uric acid)** (points 1, 55, 28, 29, 30, 31, 121 and places of pain).

- **Rheumatoid Arthritis** (points 1, 55, 120, 49, 36 and all large and small joints).

- **Paralysis of one half of the body (Hemiplegia)** (points 1, 55, 11, 12, 13, 34 or 35 and all the injured joints, massage daily).

- **Paralysis of all four limbs (Quadriplegia)** (points 1, 55, 11, 12, 13, 34,

35, 36 and all body joints and daily massage).

- **Immune system deficiency** (points 1, 55, 120, 49).

- **Muscle spasm** several dry cupping around the affected muscle.

- **Poor blood circulation** (points 1, 55, 11 and ten cups on both sides of the spine from the top to the bottom in addition to taking a teaspoon of pure organic, raw, apple cider vinegar and honey every other day).

- **Tingling arms** (points 1, 55, 40, 20, 21, arm muscles and affected joints).

- **Tingling feet** (points 1, 55, 11, 12, 13, 26, 27, feet joints and affected muscles).

- **Abdominal pain** (points 1, 55, 7, 8 and dry cupping on 137, 138, 139, 140, as well as dry cupping on the back opposite to the pain).

(Dry Cupping means without any incisions/scratches) .

Group (B)[29]

Important Note: The following points are arranged according to their importance. Sometimes, the cupping therapist does not need to use all of the points and sometimes he/she has to use them all, depending on the condition of the disease.

- **Hemorrhoids (swollen vessels around anus)** (points 1, 55, 121, 11, 6 and dry cupping on 137, 138, 139).

- **Anal Fistula (opening in skin near anus, due to formation of a channel through which**

fluid leaks) (points 1, 55, 6, 11, 12, 13 and cupping around the anus and above the fistula hole).

- **Prostate and Erectile dysfunction, ED (male impotence and urinary difficulty due to enlarged prostate gland)**(points 1, 55, 6, 11, 12, 13) and you may add for ED 125, 126, 131 on both legs, and dry cupping on 140, 143).

- **Chronic coughs and lung diseases** (points 1, 55, 4, 5, 120, 49, 115, 116, 9, 10, 117, 118, 135, 136, and two cups below both knees).

- **Hypertension (high blood pressure)** (points 1, 55, 2, 3, 11, 12, 13, 101, 32, 6, 48, 9, 10, 7, 8, and you may replace 2, 3 with 43, 44).

- **Stomach problems and ulcers** (points 1, 55, 7, 8, 50, 41, 42 and dry cupping on 137, 138, 139, 140).

- **Renal (kidney) disease** (points 1, 55, 9, 10, 41, 42 and dry cupping on 137,140).

- **Irritable bowel syndrome (abdominal cramps and discomfort characterized by bloating and trapped wind and alternating bouts of diarrhea and constipation, often related to anxiety)** (points 1, 55, 6, 48, 7, 8, 14, 15, 16, 17, 18, 45, 46 and dry cupping on 137).

- **Chronic constipation (long term difficulty with opening bowels)** (points 1, 55, 11, 12, 13, 28, 29, 30, 31).

- **Diarrhea** (dry cupping on 137, 138, 139, 140).

- **Involuntary urination (bed wetting)** (after the age of five: dry cupping on 137, 138, 139, 140, 142, 143, 125, 126).

- **Depression, withdrawal, insomnia (inability to sleep), psychological conditions and nervousness** (points 1, 55, 6, 11, 32 and below the knees).

- **Angiospasm and Arteriosclerosis (narrowing of the blood vessels due to muscular spasm or fatty deposits)**(points 1, 55, 11) (cupping points are on the places of pain in addition to a teaspoon of pure, organic, raw, apple cider vinegar and honey every other day).

- **Inflammation in the lining of the stomach (gastritis)** (points 1, 55, 121).

- **Excessive sleep** (points 1, 55, 36) in addition to a teaspoon of pure, organic, raw, apple cider vinegar and honey every other day).

- **Food allergies** (one dry cup using a light suction directly on the umbilicus pit [belly button]).

- **Sores, leg and thigh abscesses (pus filled spots) and itching of iliac fossae (itching in hip area)** (points 1, 55, 129, 120).

Group (C)[29]

Important Note: The following points are arranged according to their importance. Sometimes, the cupping therapist does not need to use all of the points and sometimes he/she has to use them all depending on the condition of the disease.

- **Heart disease** (points 1, 55, 19, 119, 7, 8, 46, 46, 47, 133, 134).

- **Diabetes** (points 1, 55, 6, 7, 8, 22, 23, 24, 25, 120, 49) note: the area of cupping should be applied with black seed oil or honey for 3 days.

- **Liver and gall bladder disease** (points 1, 55, 6, 48, 41, 42, 46, 51, 122, 123, 124 and 5 cups on the right, outer leg).

- **Varicose veins (enlarged, unsightly superficial veins) on the legs** (points 1, 55, 28, 29, 30, 31, 132 and around the veins but NOT over the veins).

- **Varicocele (enlarged unsightly veins on scrotum of male)** (points 1, 55, 6, 11, 12, 13, 28, 29, 30, 31, 125, 126).

- **Elephantiasis (swollen leg due to blockage of lymph channels)** note: the patient should rest for 2 days before cupping. He/She should also raise his/her affected leg up and then place it in warm water for two hours prior to cupping (points 1, 55, 11, 12, 13, 120, 49, 121 and around the affected leg from the top of the leg to the bottom in addition to 125, 126, 53, 54).

- **Skin diseases** (points 1, 55, 49, 120, 129, 6, 7, 8, 11 and cupping on the affected areas).

- **Overweight** (points 1, 55, 9, 10, 120, 49 and areas of desired weight loss), daily massage cupping over area of desired weight loss.

- **Underweight** (points 1, 55, 121).

- **Cellulite** daily massage cupping over affected area.

- **Infertility** (points 1, 55, 6, 11, 12, 13, 120, 49, 125, 126, 143, 41, 42).

- **Thyroid disease** (points 1, 55, 41, 42).

Group (D)[29]

- **Headaches** (points 1, 55, 2, 3) and you may replace points 2, 3 with 43, 44. If it is caused by **eye strain** add 104, 105 and 36. If it is caused by **nasal sinuses** add 102, 103 and 114. If it is caused by **high blood pressure** add 11, 101 and 32. If it is caused by **constipation** add 28, 29, 30 and 31. If it is caused by **a cold** add 120, 4 and 5. If it is caused by a**stomach ache** add 7, 8. If it is caused by **the kidneys** add 9, 10. If it is caused by **menstruation** for women add 11, 12 and 13. If it is caused by **gall bladder** and **liver** add 6, 48. If it is caused by the **spine column** perform cupping on the spine. If it is caused by tension add 6, 11 and 32. If it is caused by **anemia** add 120, 49 and take one teaspoon of black honey (molasses) with a quarter of a teaspoon of ground fenugreek and 7 ground black seeds daily. If the headache is due to **tumors** in the brain, cupping should be performed on the area of pain on the head).

- Migraine (severe headache associated with nausea and visual disturbance) (points 1, 55, 2, 3, 106 and area of pain).

- Diseases of the eyes (retina, eye disorder, blurred vision, atrophy of the eye nerves, glaucoma (Blue Water), cataract (White Water) and weak eye, eye inflammation and secretion of tears and eye sensitivity (points 1, 55, 36, 101, 104 , 105, 9, 10, 34, 35, above the eyebrows and on the hair line above the forehead).

- Tonsils, throat, gums, teeth, and the middle ear problems (dizziness, nausea and ringing in ears) (points 1, 55, 20, 21, 41, 42, 120, 49, 114, 43, 44).

- Weakness of hearing and inflammation of hearing nerve, tinnitus (ringing sensation in ears) (points 1, 55, 20, 21, 37, 38 and behind the ear).

- Nasal sinuses (points 1, 55, 102, 103, 108, 109, 36, 14 and on the hair line).

- Neuritis (inflammation) of the fifth and seventh nerves (points 1, 55, 110, 111, 112, 113, 114 and on the affected area).

- To stimulate the system of perception (encourage awareness) (points 1, 55, 2, 3, 32).

- Clinical Memory Loss (important: if point 39 is cupped unnecessarily it may cause damage to the memory. Also its unnecessary repetition may increase memory loss (point 39 occipital prominence).

- **Mute (unable to speak)** (points 1, 55, 36, 33, 107, 114).

- **To help stop smoking** (points 1, 55, 106, 11, 32).

- **Convulsion (fits)** (points 1, 55, 101, 36, 32, 107 on both sides, 114, 11, 12, 13).

- **For the treatment of mental retardation** (points 1, 55, (101 only once) 36, 32, 2, 3, 120, 49, 11, 12, 13).

- **Atrophy (loss) of brain cells (oxygen deficiency)** (points 1, 55, 101, 36, 32, 34, 35, 11 and perform cupping on the joints, muscles and neck, 43 and 44 on the front and back. Eat honey and royal jelly. Perform massage cupping daily).

Group (E)

Gynecological[29]

Important warning: pregnant women should avoid cupping during pregnancy except if they are over-due and wish to go into labour. In this case, they should have dry and massage cupping between the knee and ankle on both legs. Cupping a pregnant woman may cause miscarriage.

- **Hemorrhage (vaginal bleeding)** (points 1, 55, (3 dry cups under each breast daily until bleeding ceases).

- **Amenorrhea (absence of periods)** (points 1, 55, 129, (131 from the outside), 135, 136) .

- **Brownish Secretion** 3 dry cups under each breast daily until secretion ceases (points 1, 55, 120, 49, 11, 12, 13 and 143). If secretion has no smell, no colour or itching, perform cupping on (points 1, 55, 9, 10, 41, 42, 11, 12, 13, 143).

- **Menstruation (period) problems** (points 1, 55 (dry cupping on 125, 126, 137, 138, 139, 140, 141, 142, 143).

- **To stimulate the ovaries** (points 1, 55, 11, (dry cupping on 125, 126).

- **Pain after a uterus (womb) operation, menstrual (period) pain, the problems of ligation of the fallopian tube (tube being tied/blocked), milk existence in the breast without being** pregnant and menopausal symptoms (depression, nervousness, psychological conditions, acute uterus) (points 1, 55, 6, 48, 11, 12, 13, 120, 49) (Dry Cupping on 125, 126). To regulate the menses, it is preferred to perform cupping on the second day of the menses.

Cupping Places on Back[29]

1, the shoulder, the seventh vertebra (bone of spine) of the neck.

2 & 3, the area between the ears, the back of the head where hair grows or on the sides of the neck.

4 & 5, the air door between the two ribs upwards in the branching of the tracheae (main windpipe) and the bronchus (smaller windpipe).

6, the gall bladder at the peripheral of the right rib toward the spine.

7 & 8, on the stomach place at the middle of the back opposite to the stomach on the spinal sides.

9 & 10, the kidney centre under **7 & 8** on the middle of the back.

11, lumbar vertebrae – a prominent bone at the lower back of the vertebra column.

12 & 13, on the sides of **11,** slightly upward, 5cm away from the spine.

14, 15, 16 & 17, the colon, almost on the colon corners from the back and **18** of the middle of the spine.

19, the heart, opposite to the heart from the back and almost on the left rib side.

20 & 21, tonsils triangle that lies in the area between the neck and the shoulder with a slight bending to the back.

22 & 23, above the pancreas gland under the rib end.

24 & 25, at the beginning of the lower half of the back.

26 & 27, bilaterally at the sides of the iliac bone.

28, 29, 30 & 31, at the upper part of the buttocks.

32, on the middle of the head.

33, on the right part of the hair near the forehead or the hair line.

34 & 35, the right and left part of the brain (at the temporal sides of the brain) as well as the occipital bone.

36, the cerebellum (occipital) prominent bone on the head.

37 & 38, nearly 3cm above the ears.

39, prominent occipital bone, the deep area at the back of the head where cupping is prohibited, except in necessary cases.

40, in the middle of the back of the neck.

41 & 42, on the back of the head to the right and the left.

43 & 44, the sides of the neck.

45 & 46, nearly 3cm above the air trachea (**4-5**).

47, on the left shoulder in addition to the heart.

48, on the right rib from upward, complementary to the gall bladder knot.

49, the immunity area from the back, between the two scapulae (shoulder blades).

50, 6cm slightly above **8,** for stomach ulcers.

51 & 52, the two thigh bones (femur), from both sides.

53 & 54, the inner part of the knee from the back.

55, almost 3cm under the shoulder.

Cupping places on the face and abdomen

101, the forehead on the place of worship in praying and it is better not to repeat it.

102 & 103, above the eyebrows from the inner part of the nasal sinuses.

104 & 105, on both sides of the brows and slightly upward for headaches and sight.

106, almost 6cm above the left ear to help give up smoking.

107, nearly 4cm above the cheeks to assist in speech.

108 & 109, on the sides of the nose for nasal sinuses.

110, under the ear from the right and left.

111, 112 & 113, near the eye and the cheek and near the lip to treat the fifth and sixth nerve.

114, under the chin and it has many benefits.

115 & 116, under the ends of the clavicle (collar bone) from the outside and on the shoulders.

117 & 118, under the clavicle (collar bone) from the inside, on the chest.

119, the heart, under the middle of the left clavicle (collar bone) using four fingers of the patient himself.

120, sternum bone (breastplate), in the middle of the chest.

121, first part of the stomach directly under the chest bone.

122, 123 & 124, above the liver, right of the belly.

125 & 126, between the belly and the thigh near the pubic hair area for involuntary urination, infertility...etc.

127 & 128, on the inner part of the thighs.

129, on the back of the feet to the right.

130, on the sides of the heel from inside and outside for edema.

131, above the heel bone nearly 5cm from the outside.

132, varicocele.

133, almost 2cm above the stomach mouth and near the end of the chest bone.

134, under the left breast.

135 & 136, 5cm away from the breast nipple from the inside for the lungs.

137, 138, 139 & 140, above, right, left and under the umbilicus (belly button).

141, & 142, Right and left of **140.**

143, above the bladder.

PHARMACOLOGICAL AND PHYSIOLOGICAL ACTIONS OF CUPPING

Cupping as a complementary therapy helps many patients beyond the pain resolving treatment. There are various indications of Cupping therapy, especially joint pain, back and neck pain, arthritis, abscess, facial paralysis, and other physical health ailments. With modern technology impinging the world, cupping therapy is also transforming into a better version. A favorable balance between various vital parameters after Cupping therapy is restored by a specific mechanism. Cupping therapy helps to align the skin blood flow which is more obvious near the cupping area. It involves the removal of impure blood from superficial areas of the ailing parts. The cupping sites are more or less specific to the ailments of the patient and the number of cups varies from patient to patient, depending on the patient's condition and the cup size.[20,30]

The cupping therapy and its psychological aspect

The Damascene erudite Mohammad Amin Sheikho explained this point by saying: "Cupping is the prophets' advice" . For the whole fact, and in implementing this wholesome therapeutic art, which was recommended for application by the most honored prophets such as our masters Moses, Jesus and Mohammed (cptt) , and their followers as the savant Mohammad Amin Sheikho, the soul of the cupped-person tends to follow up those great physicians, the Physicians of the heart (soul), the inclination of the cupped-person' s soul towards them while their insights are staring incessantly at the Almighty Curing God, and there is no cure except Him, this inclination makes his soul immersed in the Almighty's Light, therefore the cupped-person' s soul is cured by the Godly Light forwarded on the prophets.[31]

Yes, cupping cures psychic ailments and ignoble characteristics and changes them into the properties of perfection. And because of detestable statuses, and before performing cupping, the cupped-person may have contracted some diseases so as that his heart is to be cured by resorting himself to God in order to attaining the recovery. Since he has followed the teachings of God as iterated by His Most Honorable Messenger; and his soul has directed itself unconsciously to its

Creator. His soul has improved and his heart has eavesdropped to the teachings of God. After that there is no need for a disease that may protect him from the evils of his spirit and of the acts for his heart has become virtuous. If the heart is reformed, the whole body becomes immuned against diseases. This psychological advantage has a great effect on recovery according to the tendency towards God. If it is strong, the cupped-person is acquitted of all diseases, and all diseases abstain protectively from attacking him.[29,31]

If the tendency towards God is feeble, the improvement is relative, but the benefit must be realized whatsoever. Cupping is all helpful. There is no harm at all in applying it. And I think the experiments on cupping for the elapsed century is enough to approve; there is no resulting harm to any person at all from applying it according to its precise rules.[29,31]

ROLE OF CUPPING THERAPY IN VARIOUS DISEASES

Medical perspective in understanding some mechanisms followed by the cupping therapy to cure or improve a number of hopeless diseases.[29-31]

1. In Splenomegaly

Splenomegalies may be due to the need of increasing the splenic work. For example, some reasons which causes these Splenomegalies are; Infectious inflammatory causes: It is believed that this kind of Splenomegaly caused by infectious inflammatory factor results from the increasing in spleen defensive activity, or due to the increasing need to refine certain compounds from the blood. And the congestive causes: this kind of Splenomegaly caused by the congestive causes results from the increase in pressure in portal circulation or in the general blood circulation. The amplification may also be due to over productivity of reticals-endothelia cells for the spleen to withdraw the spoiled cells from the blood, or due to the myeloid metaplasia, or the amplification may be due to blood rubeosis, or infiltration lesion where the spleenphagias are filled with spoiled materials which accumulated due to the effect of these diseases. It is found in this respect that the cupping therapy is a must solution for such cases (Splenomegalies). Moreover, cupping can stimulate the reticuloendothelial cells to carry out its important immunity role against germs, parasites, fungi and protozoons. It is clear that cupping application according to its rules is a secondary spleen which forms a main assistant for the spleen in the blood filtration from all unwanted materials and spoiled and dead blood cells. So cupping Medicine is a very important protective of, and curing treatment in such cases of spleen problems.

2. In Liver Diseases

When cupping removes the spoiled and senile corpuscles and the impurities from the blood, and it increases blood flow in all tissues and organs, consequently in the liver tissue. So, the liver cells will be activated and then the whole liver will be activated to perform its other functions in a complete performing. It will transform the cholesterol and the excessive triglycerides by its metabolic function, and stores the excessive sugar in blood with help from the pancreas in reducing glucose level to normal one in the diabetics. And the liver will be more active in rescuing the body from poisons, this activate all its systems including the brain and nervous system so the general health of body is better. it also heightens the regeneration of spoiled tissues in the body because the liver is responsible for the production of the necessary protein for continuation of life and growth, it is clear that cupping medicine is a cure or main improving of all hepatic problems including all types of hepatitis, and prevents from or curing the hypertension of the portal vein and all resulting dangerous problems. Prof. Dr. A. G. Jabakji, the specialist in neuromicroscopic surgery from Holland, says, "The implementation of cupping as it has been recommended is an explicit and clear entrance to complete health and good recovery. It supplies man with great power and energy by way of opening and cleaning the fine blood vessels within which blood precipitates and forms residues on its walls, and such a case is one of the causes of migraine, heart and liver diseases, and other ailments of the age." If we consider the hepatic Enzymes as a criterion for all treated cases where the levels of them are high, the findings are; after cupping they return to their normal levels.

3. Role of cupping therapy in immunity

The cupping operation increases the ability and activity of the immunity system due to the increased activity of the reticals-endothelial system, and the good blood flow through the tissues and organs heightens the immunity of the body because that the pathogens in the body are more subjected to the immunity system unites. Interferon is the quickest defensive line to be formed and secreted after the exposure of the body to any virus. Prof. Kanteel says, "That the leukocytes can produce interferon in a rate exceeding ten times more than the other body cells produce." The tests of cupping blood showed a presence of very slight rate of leukocytes in it in addition to its great effect in producing the immunity defensive cells as the phagocytes which destroy pathogenic agents. this development in the stem (initial) blood cells go toward leukocytes formation, that the case of body demanding increasing in white blood cells in order to defend the body against the pathogenic agents. Here we can say: cupping keeps the leukocytes (there is just a very slight rate of leukocytes in cupping blood) and activates its production that helps in producing interferon in abundant quantities to face the hepatic virus or cancer cells.

4. Role of cupping therapy on cardio-vascular system

In this era we hear every day about a sudden death and paralysis. These incidents are attributed to blood clots which are nothing but an agglomeration of red and white corpuscles, platelets and fibrin fibers crowded together at the ramifications of arteries to form a clot, its main happening is hypertension. In the dictionary of "Lissan Al-Arab" hyperemia means "agitation and increase," This description applies also on arterial hypertension and real increase in red corpuscles (poly Cythemia vera; Erythremia). The disturbance of the cardiac system may be caused by ischemia or oxyachrestia. Also myocardia infarction is due to ischemia resulting from arterial stenosis (arteriosclerosis) and the thrombi themselves when they are in these coronary arteries. The angina pectoris is generated when there is a decrease in supplying the heart tissue with the necessary Oxygen. Because the fat precipitations have partly blocked up the coronary artery. Then the high level of arterial hypertension may lead to complications such as: cardiac insufficiency, angina pectoris and encephala vascular incident. The long arterial hypertension may cause heart enlargement, and atherosclerosis. So, applying cupping is the best solution to prevent and treat such cases, as cupping decreases the level of fat (triglyceride, cholesterol) in blood to normal one, gets rid of hypertension and increases the blood flow through heart tissue after cleaning the arteries and preventing them from atherosclerosis.

5. Effect of cupping therapy on digestive system

The blood stagnation in the veins of the stomach and the intestines destroys their secretive and absorption functions and that will lead to severe bleeding, especially the vessels of the stomach, the intestines, the esophagus and the rectum, and blood clots in the legs and feet, hemorrhoids, and severe menstruation "in women", all of what mentioned above leads blood pressure to go down. So, cupping medicine activates the blood flow and consequently prevents blood from the in the digestive system. Therefore we cupping prevents and treats all the above mentioned cases. Most patients have their problems with hemorrhoids come to an end after performing cupping. The heightening blood pressure with a sluggish blood circulation leads to harm the biliary tracts and increases the density of the bile. Here cholesterol and bilirubin start to crystallize and that hinders the circulation of the arterial blood. Whereas the compactness of the aged red corpuscles and their precipitation result in the impeded circulation in portal vein. Eventually, the tension of the portal vein heightens to push a part of the blood to the peripheral circulation round the liver through vessels anastomosis, consequently the spleen congests and enlarges and also does the venous vessels in the pancreas leading to its atrophy and its inability to do its functions. This is what we have seen. In fact, the cupping therapy is a prevention and cure for all these problems and saves us from the trouble.

6. Effect of cupping therapy on nervous system

The vascular incidents of the brain can be referred to two things: • The ischemia and its rate (80%). • Bleeding and its rate (20%). If the ischemia extends, it will lead to brain congestion and results in hemiplegia. And this what we have avoided its occurrence by performing a cupping operation. The cupping operation is helpful in regulating the blood coming to the brain. It is also found to be useful in cases of memory weakness and lack of concentration. It also helps in controlling and regulating feelings and affections. . Cupping was also mentioned for its usefulness for epilepsy and in improving the hearing if the cause was ischemia, and the stability resulting from lack of the coming blood.

7. The Effect of Cupping Operation on Diabetes

One of the factors of heightening the rate of sugar in blood is ischemic the case where the body is stimulated to liberate glucose in order to raise the activity of its organs. Unluckily, the cause is not in the burning or in the ability, but the ischemic meager. And this explains the secret of immediate recovery for diabetic people soon after performing the therapy. The activity of the liver and pancreas share much in reducing the level of sugar in the blood. This is what we have seen while performing the operation.

8. The Effect of Cupping Operation on the Eye Diseases

Cupping, while playing its role in removing from the blood all that impedes its movement and prevents it from stagnation. In this way, it activates the blood circulation and improves the perfusion of tissues and organs, and at the same time, it raises the activities of the various organs and systems of the body in addition to what result from the rearrangement of the hormone secretion leading to raise the immunity and defense of the body and its systems, especially the brain, the optic nerve, and the retina improving, in his way, the general state of the eyesight.

9. The Effect of Cupping therapy on the Kidneys

The two kidneys usually do their duty of cleaning the body from nitrogen products, regulate the concentration of sodium, and metabolize the body liquids. They also concentrate the ions in blood and the balance of PH in the body, the deficiency of blood perfusion to the kidneys breaks down the kidneys from doing their elimination function and that may cause kidney failure, or to fall victim of Boliva disease which affects the brain and kills its cells. Cupping eliminates the ischemia from the kidneys and encourages them to function their duties to the best and that will increase the resistance of the body against diseases in general.

APPLICATION METHOD OF CUPPING TREATMENT

The cupping- practitioner prepares the papers clips and wraps them in the form of funnel cones taken from newspaper for easiness of burning and in the morning of the day of cupping application:

1) The wishful person in cupping takes off his upper clothes and keeps his back naked after warming the room with a stove in order to make the surroundings warm (if it is not already warm). It is better to provide moderate warmth rather than hotness.

2) The person sits cross-legged, or sits in the way he could rest his body. Any way, he must sit somehow straight up.

3) The practitioner lights a candle and fixes it near him. Then he puts on sterile medical gloves on his hands to start work.

4) After sterilizing the skin region very well, the practitioner holds one cup in his right hand and the other hand holds a small conical paper and lights it from the candle. When the piece of paper burns well. He inserts it quickly inside the cup, and fixes the cup quickly and lightly on the back in the two places, the right one and the left one.

5) The work requires lightness and quickness of hand which the practitioner acquires by practice. The operation is easy and facile. Then he holds another cup and in the same way he fixes it in a symmetrical place of the first one. He must be sure of the fixing force of two cups on the body and their pulling force on the skin. If the two cups are not strongly fixed, the practitioner must take off the weak cup and empty it from the ash and the rest of the burned cone, and then he repeats the procedure by burning another cone of paper, puts it inside the cup while it is at its utmost burning and fixing the cup on the same place.

Important Remarks: If there is hair on the back (the cupping place) of the person, the cupping-performer must only shave it with a razor in the limited symmetrical places for the two cups in order to fix them firmly on the body. Otherwise their adhesion with the skin will not be complete, the air can infiltrate into the cups and the adhesive force of both cups fails. The practitioner must keep the burning cone away from the opening of the cup lest it becomes hot and, in turn, it burns the skin a little on fixing it. When the practitioner repeats the fixation or refrains from doing it due to a weak fixation, he must change the cup for another one because the defect may be from the cup itself (due to a crack in it, or its edge is not regular, so the air gets through the cup). The most important thing is that the pull of both cups must be strong enough in order to get the best use of cupping.

6) The practitioner must wait for (2-3) minutes letting the two cups to fix themselves on the back of the person. Then he takes off the first cup and empties it from the remains of the burned cone of paper and repeats fixing it by burning another paper cone. Likewise, he takes off the other cup,

after fixing the first one, and re-fixes it as quickly as possible in order to prevent the congested blood from going away.

Remark: For removing the cup from the body, we always resort to holding it by putting its belly between the thumb and the forefinger of one hand and at the same time by putting the other one on the body of the person on the upper part of his back adjacent to the mouth of the cup, and we press it on the skin while the holding hand pulls the cup downward from its belly by removing the upper edge and keeping the lower edge stuck on the body. When we remove the upper edge, the air fills in the cup and eventually we can easily remove the cup and put it away from the body of the person.

7) After the elapse of (2 - 3 minutes), we repeat removing the two cups and fixing them again (and these repetitions (twice) are made in order not to let the pull weaken in time).

8) During the last fixation (the last one) of the cups (in case the practitioner finds that the fixation of the two cups is weak and he cannot strengthen them, he repeats the fixation for a fourth time). He starts in sterilizing the blade very well, or it may already be sterilized, and puts it in a piece of cotton wetted with antiseptic solution right from the beginning of his work.

9) Then he lightly and quickly removes the first cup and disinfects its place with antiseptics or with sterilizing spray, and holds the angle of the blade in his hand, between the thumb and the forefinger,

and slits the skin in superficial slashes apart (0.5 – 1 cm) from each other. He cuts few slashes up and down mentioning the name of God from the beginning of his work.

10) When he finishes the slight slashes in the first place, he fixes the cup on it slightly and quickly. Then the cup starts sucking the spoiled blood. Then the practitioner removes the second cup, disinfects its place and repeats the act of slashing and re-fixes it in former place.

Important Remark The blade is to be used for one person exclusively, and then it should be thrown away in the wastebasket. It must never be used for another person even if it is disinfected with antiseptics.

11) When the practitioner removes the last two cups, he must disinfect their places (the slight cuts) very well, and must put a piece of sterilized gauze sprinkled with a disinfectant solution by means of an atomizer on place of the cuts.

12) After the cupping therapy, the person can eat a dish of "fat' toush" the ingredients of which and its way of preparation have already explained, or he may eat a meal of vegetable salad...

13) I want to recapitulate in here: it is forbidden for the cupped-person to drink milk or eat any dairy products all the day and its night only (for twenty-four hours) in which he has performed the cupping operation because milk contains calcium and some amino acids which lead to disturbances in blood pressure.

14) The cups must be cleaned and disinfected very well soon after the operation if possible, or they must be destroyed completely in a special place for rubbish.

Important Remark: It is forbidden for the cupped-person to drink milk or eat any dairy products such as cheese, yogurt and cream, or eat any meal cooked in these kinds of dairy products during the day of cupping, i.e. only the day of cupping and its night because milk and its derivatives mostly lead to nausea and evoke vomiting, and make disturbances in blood pressure; all that may lead to harm and some health problems.

PATIENTS INFORMATION

What to expect?

Remember that Hijama is an easy yet very effective way of assisting your body to heal or prevent it from becoming imbalanced and consequently unwell. The therapist will show you a cup (there are different sizes of cups available, we will choose one that is appropriate for you) that will be placed either on the area/s of pain or on specific points of your body to promote healing or detoxification. We use disposable cups brand new, after using it on one patient we obviously get rid of it. We do not use glass cups with fire (also known as fire cupping) because No.1 accidents can happen and we do not want to end up burning our patients No.2 glass cups needs to be sterilized very well with good sterilizing tools, so just to be on the safe side we do not use glass cups. Everything we use is brand new from the pack. Remember the cuts are very light scratches, and nothing is going in as the suction is always pulling out, this is a smart therapy, your skin filters/fights bacteria and other pathogens every day, so the chance of getting seriously infected is very low, especially when combined with the health and hygiene standard procedure.[29]

Preparation before and after treatment[29]

Before:

The best advice is to fast; however, some people are unwell or feel very weak when fasting. It is better not to eat solid food for at least 2-3 hours before treatment so that the body is not occupied with digesting food. It is best to eat healthy food 24 hours before and after treatment. You are allowed to drink water!

After:

After the hijama session try to rest as some people feel very tired and need to relax or sleep. Others feel energised as they physically and psychologically feel refreshed; but do not exert yourself even if you feel like this. Do not underestimate the treatment and remember to respect the fact that your body needs rest in order to replenish and repair. Keep warm; do not allow the areas that have been treated to be exposed to the wind, water or cold. This also means no showers or baths for the next 2 hours. Try not to eat red meat and dairy products for the next 24 hours. This is because these items take up 40% of your body' s energy to digest, and this energy is needed to rejuvenate your body after having the treatment.

Reminder: If you plan to do hijama on your head please shave your hair before coming to the hijama premises. No blade zero or blade one, please shave properly with a razor blade. The cup becomes very difficult to place and to create a negative pressure becomes very hard as the hair prevents it from creating a suction. Also if you sweat a lot please have a shower before coming to the hijama premises for health and hygiene reasons.

FREQUENTLY ASKED QUESTIONS (FAQS)

What is Cupping Therapy (Hijama)?

Hijama comes from the root word 'al-hajm' , which simply means "sucking" . Cupping is the modern term for this ancient form of medical treatment in which a partial vacuum is created in cups that are positioned onto the surface of the body. The vacuum created by either heat or suction draws up skin, subcutaneous tissue and muscle layers a few millimetres into the cups. Cupping therapy now practised for over a thousand years is where a local suction is applied on the skin. The pressure of the suction causes dispels stagnant blood and lymph fluid, causing it to mobilize and flow, this promotes healing at the the site and surrounding areas. The suction that is used can be created by a professional suction machine, fire or other handheld vacuum devices.

What is History of Cupping Treatment/therapy?

Cupping treatment commonly referred to as Hijama, has been around for thousands of years, and developed over time from the original use of hollowed out animal horns to suck out and drain the toxins out of snakebites and skin lesions. Horns slowly evolved into bamboo cups, which were eventually replaced by glass. Therapeutic applications evolved with the refinement of the cup itself, and with the cultures that employed cupping as a health care technique.

The true origin of cupping treatment still remains uncertain to this day. Some consider the Chinese to be responsible for cupping. The earliest recorded use of cupping treatment from the famous alchemist and herbalist, Ge Hong (281-341 A.D.), which incorporates the popular saying "Acupuncture and cupping, more than half of the ills cured."

The Chinese expanded the utilization of cupping to include its use in surgery to divert blood flow from the surgery site. By the 19th century, after much extensive research, a collaborative effort between the former Soviet Union and China confirmed the clinical efficacy of cupping therapy. Since then, cupping has become a mainstay of government-sponsored hospitals of Traditional Chinese medicine (TCM).

The earliest record of pictorial record of cupping was discovered in Egypt around 1500 B.C. Translations of the hieroglyphic text about ancient medicine detailed the use of cupping for conditions such as fever, pain, vertigo, menstrual imbalances, weakened appetites and accelerating the "healing crisis" of disease. From the Egyptians, cupping was introduced to the ancient Greeks, where Hippocrates, the Father of Modern Medicine, recommended the use of cups for a variety of disorders such angina and menstrual irregularities.

Q. What are typical Cupping sessions?

A. Every 7-21 days usually for 6-8 sessions, depending on condition, age, efficiency of body's circulatory system. Varies person to person depending temperament of the personality.

Q. How long is a typical Cupping session?

A. A session of just cups lasts 15-30 minutes. When combined as a part of the treatment with acupuncture or massage it can be up to an hour.

Q. How does Cupping work?

A. Cupping causes the tissues beneath the cup to be drawn up and swell, and an increase in blood flow to the affected area. This enhanced blood flow under the cup draws impurities and toxins away from the nearby tissues and organs to the skin, from where they are expelled. The release of the vacuum redirects "toxic" blood that had pooled at the site and redirects it to other areas of the body, thus allowing "fresh" blood to replace it. This facilitates the healing process. Localised and deep-tissue healing takes place. Cupping diverts toxins and impurities from important organs – such as the liver or kidney – to the less important organ, the skin. In dry cupping, the toxins are brought to the underlying skin; in wet cupping the toxins are brought out of the body, onto the surface of the skin.

Q. Is cupping a cure for every disease?

Cupping is a cure for every disease if performed in its correct time. The Messenger (p.b.u.h) said, "Indeed in cupping there is a cure." [Saheeh Muslim (5706)].

The Messenger(p.b.u.h) said, "Whoever performs cupping on the 17th, 19th or 21st day (of the Islamic month) then it is a cure for every disease." [Saheeh Sunan Abi Dawud (3861)].

There are specific 13 points on the body where the cups are applied for each ailment.

Q. Is cupping from the Sunnah?

Above are just some of the authentic narrations which show that cupping is from the Sunnah

of the Messenger.(p.b.u.h). The Messenger (p.b.u.h) said, "Whoever revives a Sunnah from my Sunnah and the people practise it, s/he will have the same reward of those who practise it without their reward diminishing" [Sunan ibn Maajah (209)].

Q. Cupping Is The Best of Remedies?

Anas ibn Maalik (may Allah be pleased with him) reported that the Messenger (p.b.u.h) said, "Indeed the best of remedies you have is cupping" [Saheeh al-Bukhaaree (5371)].

Abu Hurairah (may Allaah be pleased with him) reported that the Messenger (p.b.u.h) said, "If there was something excellent to be used as a remedy then it is cupping." [Saheeh Sunan abi Dawud (3857), Saheeh Sunan ibn Maajah (3476).

Q. The Angels Recommending Cupping?

Abdullah ibn Abbas (may Allaah be pleased with him) reported that the Messenger (p.b.u.h) said, "I did not pass by an angel from the angels on the night journey except that they all said to me: Upon you is cupping, O Muhammad."[Saheeh Sunan ibn Maajah (3477)]. In the narration reported by Abdullah ibn Mas'ud (may Allah be pleased with him) the angels said, "Oh Muhammad, order your Ummah (nation) with cupping."

Q. Cupping Is A Prevention?

Anas ibn Maalik (May Allah be pleased with him) reported that the Messenger (p.b.u.h) said, "Whoever wants to perform cupping then let him search for 17th, 19th and 21st and let none of you allow his blood to rage (boil) such that it kills him." [Saheeh Sunan ibn Maajah (3486)].

Anas ibn Maalik (may Allaah be pleased with him) reported that the Messenger (p.b.u.h) said, "When the weather becomes extremely hot, seek aid in cupping. Do not allow your blood to rage (boil) such that it kills you." [Reported by Hakim in his 'Mustadrak' and he authenticated it and Imam ad-Dhahabi agreed (4/212)].

Q. In Cupping There Is A Cure and A blessing?

Abdullah ibn Abbas (May Allah be pleased with him) reported that the Messenger (p.b.u.h) said, "Healing is in three things: in the incision of the cupper, in drinking honey, and in cauterizing with fire, but I forbid my Ummah (nation) from cauterization (branding with fire)." [Saheeh al-Bukhaaree (5681), Saheeh Sunan ibn Maajah (3491)].

Jaabir ibn Abdullah (may Allaah be pleased with him) reported that the Messenger (p.b.u.h) said,

"Indeed in cupping there is a cure." [Saheeh Muslim (5706)].

Ibn Umar (may Allaah be pleased with him) reported that the Messenger (p.b.u.h) said, "Cupping on an empty stomach is best. In it is a cure and a blessing..."[Saheeh Sunan ibn Maajah (3487)].

'Alaa Ar-Reeq in arabic means to fast until after being treated with cupping. Once the treatment of cupping has been completed, one may eat and drink.

Q. Cupping In Its Time Is A Cure For Every Disease?

Abu Hurairah (may Allaah be pleased with him) reported that the Messenger (p.b.u.h) said,

"Whoever performs cupping on the 17th, 19th or 21st day (of the Islamic, lunar month) then it is a cure for every disease." [Saheeh Sunan abi Dawud (3861)].

Q. The Best Days For Cupping?

The best days for cupping are the 17th, 19th and 21st of the Islamic month which coincide with Monday, Tuesday or Thursday. Anas ibn Maalik (may Allaah be pleased with him) reported that the Messenger (p.b.u.h) said, "Whoever wants to perform cupping then let him search for 17th, 19th and 21st day. [Saheeh Sunan ibn Maajah (3486)].

Ibn Umar (may Allaah be pleased with him) reported that the Messenger (p.b.u.h) said, "Cupping on an empty stomach* is best. In it is a cure and a blessing. It improves the intellect and the memory. So cup yourselves with the blessing of Allaah on Thursday. Perform cupping on Monday and Tuesday for it is the day that Allaah saved Ayoub from a trial. He was inflicted with the trial on Wednesday. You will not find leprosy except (by being cupped) on Wednesday or Wednesday night." [Saheeh Sunan ibn Maajah (3487)].

As for the Islamic day and night, the night enters before the day. So at sunset on Tuesday, Wednesday night comes in. Cupping is best performed during the daytime between the adhaan of fajr and the adhaan of maghrib because yawm in arabic means daytime. The Sunnah days for cupping every month are when the 17th or 19th or 21st of the lunar month coincide with a Monday,

Tuesday or Thursday. These are the best and most beneficial days for cupping. If one is not able to be cupped on 17th, 19th or 21st (coinciding with Monday, Tuesday or Thursday) then any Monday, Tuesday or Thursday of the month.

Q. Are you going to pump out all of my blood?

Relax! The blood that comes out is from the surface of the skin, it is not from the mainstream. If you are thinking your blood system only contains hemoglobin, platelets, plasma and white blood cells you are wrong, there are so many other junks that fly around in your body such as dead blood cells, blood clots, different toxins and pathogen. Different people's body give different responses, sometimes hardly anything comes out from a person's skin and that is a good thing. Because the cuts are very light the body heals the area very quick and automatically the blood stops coming out. We constantly analyze the patient if they are feeling well or not. Only in paradise you will be 100% pure and clean.

Q. How long does it take to do hijama?

Depends how many cups you do, the standard five cups on the back takes approximately 15 mins.

Q. How often should I do hijama?

It is totally up to you, some do it every month as a preventative medicine in the sunnah days, which is 17th, 19th and the 21st of the Islamic lunar calender. For non-veg.4 months d for vegetarian 6 months or even after a year depends. Hijama is a detoxification therapy, there are other detox programs that people follow for example, they may start to have more (organic) fruits and vegetables, antioxidant drinks, cut down on fatty unhealthy foods and soon.

Q. What are benefits of Cupping Therapy?

A. Benefits of cupping therapy are:

- ❖ Colds & Influenza
- ❖ Headaches
- ❖ Arthritis
- ❖ Intercostal Neuralgia
- ❖ Intestinal disorders
- ❖ Sciatica
- ❖ Rheumatism
- ❖ High blood pressure

❖ Bronchial asthma & congestion

❖ Gynecological disorders

❖ Kidney disorders (including frequent/urgent urination)

❖ Dispels colds and respiratory infections

❖ Relieves gastrointestinal symptoms such as stomachache, vomiting and diarrhea

❖ Liver disorders

❖ Gallbladder disorders

❖ Dermatological Disorders such as pigmentation imbalance

❖ Depression

❖ Fibromyalgia & Chronic Fatigue Syndrome

❖ Anxiety & insomnia

❖ Post-injury trauma

❖ Post-surgery adhesions

❖ Cellulite

❖ Musculo-skeletal problems: pain, spasms, cramps, tightness, numbness, stiffness of the back and neck

❖ Chronic gastric pain

❖ Vertigo

❖ Menopausal discomforts

❖ Activates the skin, clears stretch marks and wrinkles

Q. Is there anything I should do, or not do after a cupping treatment?

A. As with any kind of deep tissue work, be sure to drink plenty of water after your session to flush the flotsam and jetsam that have been release by your tissues. It is best not do any kind of strenuous physical activity immediately after your session, nor should you engage in delirious amounts of alcohol or an ice cream binge. Ideally, give yourself an afternoon or evening' s worth of time to allow yourself to soak in the gentle feelings of glide and ease that are the result of your muscles and blood being on good speaking terms.

Q. What are Safety concerns during cupping?

A. The following safety aspects should be adhered to by the cupping practitioner:

- ❖ The practitioner must wear disposable latex gloves whilst carrying out both types of cupping.
- ❖ The cups used must be thoroughly sterilised immediately before use.

❖ Before cupping actually begins, the patient ·s blood pressure and pulse must be checked.

❖ The blades used for wet cupping incisions should be disposable.

❖ The incisions in wet cupping should be superficial, involving the epidermis only.

❖ An antiseptic cream should be applied to the incisions after cupping is terminated.

❖ The patient should be questioned on how he or she feels – any unusual sensation or fever.

❖ All other necessary safety measures should be in place.

Q. What are contraindications during cupping therapy?

A. Cupping is contraindicated in cases of severe diseases, such as:

❖ Cardiac failure, renal failure, ascites due to hepato-cirrhosis and severe edema, as well as hemorrhagic diseases such as allergic pupura, hemophilia and leukemia, and clients with dermatosis, destruction of skin, or allergic dermatitis.

❖ Cupping should not be applied on an area where a hernia exists or has occurred in the past.

❖ For pregnant women, work on the lower abdomen, inner side of the leg and sacral (tail bone) region should be avoided. Also, if you have never received a cupping treatment, you should wait until the 2nd trimester to receive your first treatment.

Other contraindications:

- ❖ Broken bones

- ❖ Dislocations

- ❖ Slipped disks

- ❖ Those undergoing cancer treatments such as radiation

- ❖ Sunburn

- ❖ Ruptured, ulcerated, inflamed skin

- ❖ Fever-

- ❖ Bleeding disorders

- ❖ Acute stages of Psoriasis, Eczema, or Rosacea

- ❖ Dehydration

Warnings:

If you are on blood thinners, are a hemophiliac, diabetic, or have high or low blood pressure, shorter, lighter techniques are recommended and must be used for your overall wellness. Those with low blood pressure should warn the therapist ahead of time as you'll need extra time to rest before rising after a treatment and accommodations will need to be made.

REFERENCES:

1. J. Turk, E. Allen. Bleeding and cupping, Ann R Coll Surg Engl, 65 (1983), pp. 128–131

2. H. Christopoulou-Aletra, N. Papavramidou. Cupping: an alternative surgical procedure used by hippocratic physicians, J Altern Complement Med, 14 (2008), pp. 899–902

3. R. Huber, M. Emerich, M. Braeunig. Cupping - is it reproducible? Experiments about factors determining the vacuum. Complement Ther Med, 19 (2011), pp. 78–83

4. K. Farhadi, D. Schwebel, M. Saeb, M. Choubsaz, R. Mohammadi, A. Ahmadi. The effectiveness of wet-cupping for nonspecific low back pain in Iran: a

randomized controlled trial. Complement Ther Med, 17 (2009), pp. 9–15

5. A. Michalsen, S. Bock, R. Ludtke, et al. Effects of traditional cupping therapy in patients with carpal tunnel syndrome: a randomized controlled trial. J Pain, 10 (2009), pp. 601–608

6. Moetaz El-Domyati, F. Saleh, M. Barakat, N. Mohamed. Evaluation of cupping therapy in some dermatoses. Egyptian Dermatol Online J, 9 (2013), pp. 1–15

7. N. Anjum, S. Jamil, A. Hannan, J. Akhtar, B. Ahmad. Clinical efficacy of Hijamat (Cupping) in Waja-ul-Mafasil (Arthritis). Indian J Tradit Knowl, 4 (2005), pp. 412–415

8. W. Brockbank. The ancient art of cupping. J Chin Med, 21 (1986), pp. 22–25

9. A. Al-Bedah, M. Khalil, A. Elolemy, I. Elsubai, A. Khalil. Hijama (Cupping): a review of the evidence Foc Altern Complement Ther, 16 (2011), pp. 12–16

10. L. Stovner, K. Hagen, R. Jensen, et al. The global burden of headache: a documentation of headache prevalence and disability worldwide Cephalalgia, 27 (2007), pp. 193–210

11. I. Chirali. Cupping Therapy: Traditional Chinese Medicine. (1st ed.)Elsevier Health Sciences, London (1999)

12. M. Teut, S. Kaiser, M. Ortiz, et al. Pulsatile dry cupping in patients with osteoarthritis of the knee–

a randomized controlled exploratory trial. BMC Complement Altern Med, 12 (2012), pp. 1–9

13. K. Al-Rubaye, The clinical and histological skin changes after the cupping therapy (Al-Hijamah). J Turk Acad Dermatol, 6 (2012), pp. 1–7

14. M. Mahdavi, T. Ghazanfari, M. Aghajani, F. Danyali, M. Naseri. Evaluation of the effects of traditional cupping on the biochemical, haematological and immunological factors of human venous blood. A. Bhattacharya (Ed.), A Compendium of Essays on Alternative Therapy, InTech, Croatia (2012), pp. 67–88

15. H. Cao, Li Xun, J. Liu. An updated review of the efficacy of cupping therapy. PLOS ONE, 7 (2012), pp. 1–14

16. J. Dearlove, A. Verguei, N. Birkin, P. Latham. An anachronistic treatment for asthma. Br Med J, 283 (1981), pp. 1684–1685

17. G. Blaser, K. Santos, U. Bode, H. Vetter, A. Simon. Effect of medical honey on wounds colonised or infected with MRSA. J Wound Care, 16 (2007), pp. 325–328

18. S. El Sayed, H. Mahmoud, M. Nabo. Methods of wet cupping therapy (Al-Hijamah): in light of modern medicine and prophetic medicine. Altern Integ Med, 2 (2013), pp. 1–16

19. S. Ahmed, N. Madbouly, S. Maklad, E. Abu-Shady. Immuno modulatory effects of blood - letting cupping therapy in patients with

rheumatoid arthritis. Egypt J Immunol, 12 (2005), pp. 39–51

20. M. Bilal, R. Khan, A. Ahmed, S. Afroz. Partial evaluation of technique used in cupping therapy. J Basic Appl Sci, 7 (2011), pp. 65–68

21. N. Iqbal, A. Ansari. Al-Hijamah (Cupping): the natural holistic healing art–a review. Int J Adv Ayurveda, Yoga, Unani, Siddha, Homeopathy, 2 (2013), pp. 23–30

22. H. Cao, M. Han, X. Li, et al. Clinical research evidence of cupping therapy in China: a systematic literature review. BMC Complement Altern Med, 10 (2010), pp. 1–10

23. Y. Tian, G. Wang, T. Huang, S. Jia, Y. Zhang, W. Zhang. Impacts on skin blood flow under moving

cupping along meridians in different directions. Zhongguo Zhen Jiu, 33 (2013), pp. 247–251

24. Y. Jung, J. Kim, H. Lee, et al. A herpes simplex virus infection secondary to acupuncture and cupping. Ann Dermatol, 23 (2011), pp. 67–69

25. J. Lu, X. Chu, L. Wang, W. Tang, Y. Zhou, P. Sun.The change of negative pressure in the cupping-cup and its influence on the depth of filiform-needle insertion. Sheng Wu Yi Xue Gong Cheng Xue Za Zhi, 27 (2010), pp. 71–74

26. M. Lee, J. Kim, J. Kong, D. Lee, B. Shin. Developing and validating a sham cupping device Acupunct Med, 28 (2010), pp. 200–204. View Record in Scopus | Full Text via CrossRef | Citing articles (8)

27. Z. Hong,Clinical application sliding cupping. J Chin Med, 67 (2001), pp. 38–39

28. S. El Sayed, A. Al-quliti, H. Mahmoud, et al. Therapeutic benefits of Al-Hijamah: in light of modern medicine and prophetic medicine. Am J Med Biol Res, 2 (2014), pp. 46–71

29. H.Izharul. Encyclopedia of cupping therapy.2nd edition, CS Publication,USA

30. Piyush Mehta, Vividha Dhapte. Cupping therapy: A prudent remedy for a plethora of medical ailments.Sciencedirect.com/science/article

31. A.K john Aliayas, Mohammad Amino Sheikho. Cupping: A prophetical medicine appears in its new scientific perspective.

Cupping Therapy Pictures

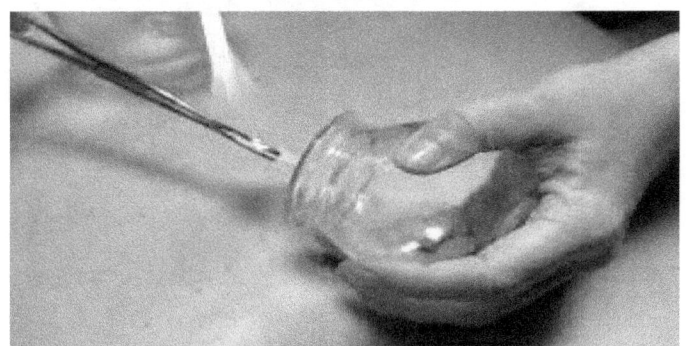

Pic 1: Fire Cupping

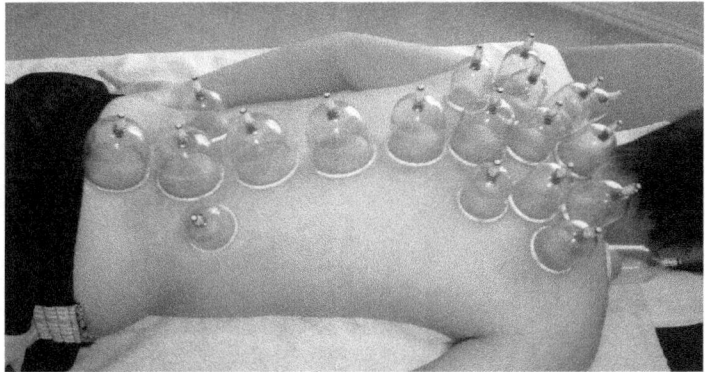

Pic 2: Dry Cupping

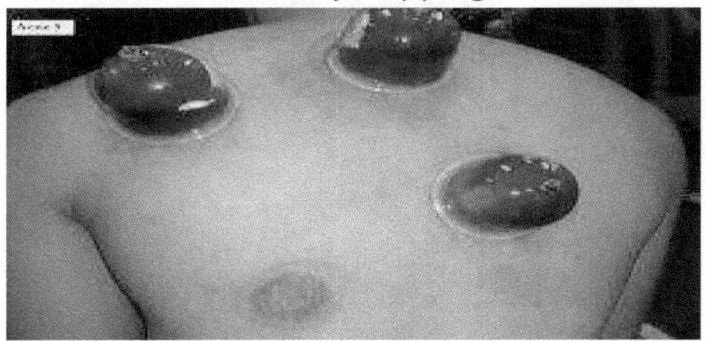

Pic 3: Wet Cupping

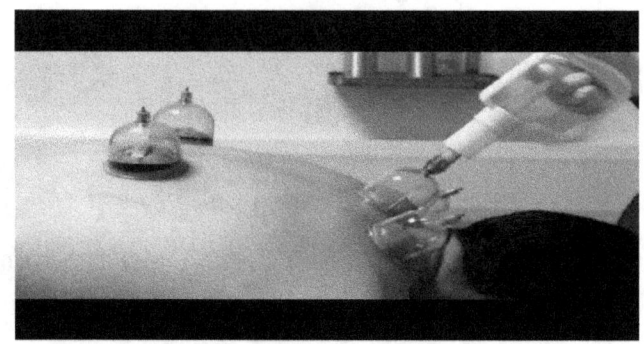

Pic 4: Performing Wet Cupping

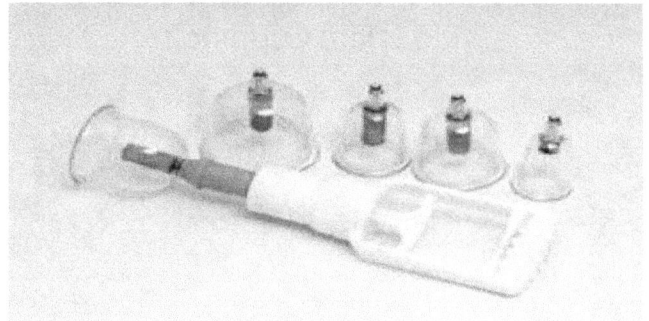

Pic 5: Cupping Pump and Cups

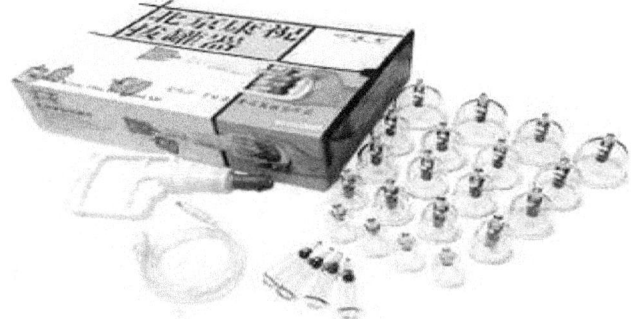

Pic 6: Cupping Box

THANKS YOU

www.ingramcontent.com/pod-product-compliance
Lightning Source LLC
Chambersburg PA
CBHW070814180526
45168CB00002B/623